ABC's of THCBD:
A Study of Cannabis; Its History and Uses

DOUGLAS FOX II

Copyright © 2018 Douglas Fox II

All rights reserved.

ISBN: 9781728993980
ISBN-13:

DEDICATION

For my loving wife Cheryl, family and you..

CONTENTS

	Introduction	i
1	A: Account	1
	When the tide Turned	Pg 4
2	B: Brief	Pg 7
	What are Cannabinoids?	Pg 9
	Terpenes	Pg 11
	ECS	Pg 12
	It's Alphabet Soup	Pg 14
3	C: Consumption	Pg 20
	Inhaling	Pg 21
	Ingesting	Pg 22
	Topical	Pg 23
4	Final Note	Pg 25
	References	Pg 30

INTRODUCTION

This book is one in a string of journeys I would have never guessed to take had you asked three years ago. It started with my mother's passing from cancer, and how we tried to help ease her pain. Had it not been for that experience, I would not have found myself immersed in the world of cannabis (full disclosure: we own and operate a cannabis processing facility). Without the tireless efforts of every researcher listed in my reference list, I would have nothing to show. Without our customers and their consumers, I would have no reason to tell what I have compiled; What I believe through my own research is the real story behind Cannabis. The idea for writing this book started by asking a dispensary's intake manager how we could help. The more dispensaries we visited, the more we found a need for a single authoritative point of information that could be passed on to customers that answered the most basic, pressing question: *"My doctor told me to buy some weed to help with my [fill in the blank], and I'm new to pot; what should I choose?"*. Budtenders usually have a cornucopic collection of cannabis facts and trivia in their heads; a very professional attitude, and a true love of helping customers. What they typically don't have, is enough time to explain the different ways you can use cannabis, or how each method of consumption can affect you; and so, this book was born to fill in the gaps. Before we get into the meat and potatoes of cannabis use, I offer these thoughts:

- *One:* Whether you call it hemp, pot, weed, ganja, or one of many other slang names, recognize that it's all cannabis. It is time to bring this plant in all its forms, out from under the bed and sock drawer and back into the light as a legitimate tool for healing.

- *Two* (baby-boomers take head): Today's cannabis has increased in potency from the 60's and 70's. Why? Because growers have been selectively breeding high THC producing plants and leaving the lower ones to fall away; much like selectively breeding dogs for specific purposes (Lafrance, 2015). The average cannabis plant now is higher THC producing than before, as the ability to grow legitimately has forced the desire to increase quality. Means the odds of you getting a 'lower quality high' are less than before (Miller, 2017).

- *Three*: There's real science and statistical data proving cannabis' health benefits. Terms like *synergy,* and *the Entourage Effect* that used to be treated as dubious claims are finding real traction in the medical and scientific world. If you're not familiar with either, think peanut butter and jelly. Each is good on its own, but together they make a much better sandwich. Research shows it takes more than one cannabinoid or terpene to maximize the benefits your body can absorb from cannabis, but don't get caught up in whether to choose isolates over whole-plant extracts, ratios, or amounts of terpenes and cannabinoids in products; each person's tolerance level and needs are different. Where one person might be able to eat half a brownie and not be affected, another might be stuck on the couch (referred to as couch-lock) for hours from the same dose (Renee, 2005). Treat cannabis with respect; learn to start low and slow (called *micro-dosing*), then gradually work up to the level your body needs and can handle. Although no one in recorded history has ever died directly from a cannabis overdose, a side effect of taking too high a dosage of THC for some can be acute anxiety or paranoia; very unwelcome and disturbing feelings (Wing, 2017). I highly recommend watching Bill Engvall's YouTube video on getting stoned for the first time. An amazing comedian; go to YouTube and look up "We Got the Stone Show 2018". He says volumes in a short skit about the importance of how *not* to use cannabis for the first time.

- *Four*. The scientific and anecdotal data I am passing on comes from reputable researchers; doctors, scientists and field specialists that have been studying the benefits of cannabis for years; even the Wikipedia information comes with a plethora of references. The truth about cannabis has been known and appreciated for centuries; the common threads between all these researchers? One; it works. Two, cannabis is not something to fear, just respected. By passing on these references and findings, I hope it helps to shed some light and dispel the stereotypes and biases associated with cannabis. May you find this an easy and enlightening read; one that helps make your choices simpler on your path to relief and a better quality of life.

A: ACCOUNT
SOME HISTORY SURROUNDING CANNABIS

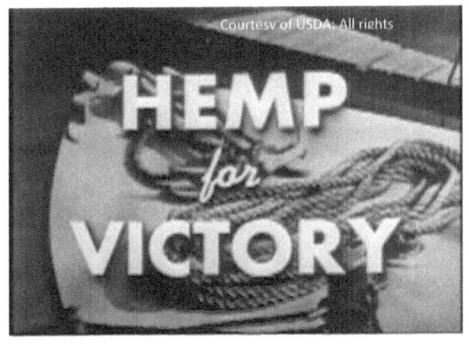

Cannabis is one of the older known plants to mankind; recorded as domesticated around 3500 BCE, two thousand years after cereals [like oatmeal] (Hirst, 2018). For over 12,000 years it has been a major part of our collective consciousness (Sawler et al, 2015), and has always played a major role in our industrialized world; grown as a required cash crop in our original colonies (Abel, 1980, & Wikipedia, 2018), then fast forward to World War II, the U.S. Agricultural Department did its utmost to develop the hemp market to better supply our military needs and quickly depleting reserves, previously attained from the far-East [1][2][4][5][6]. It has only been in the last 100 years that cannabis has become a 'blight' upon mankind, and only since 1970 it has been considered a 'toxic plant with no benefit' [6]. Cannabis has been used to make paper, rope, clothing, sails, shoes, even fuel, and of course medicinal oils and teas throughout history (Abel, 1980), but suddenly was being included into the war on heroin, cocaine and other addictive drugs (Wikipedia, 2018). The Volstead Act [Prohibition] had recently been repealed, but there was still a very large conservative segment of the population that believed very strongly in the concept that our world could be made better by eliminating the use of all addictive drugs [1][2][4][5][6]. It has been documented that Mr. Anslinger chose to ignore the medical communities' recommendations and even earlier studies, like the United Kingdom's House of Commons Indian Hemp Drug Commission Report of 1893; where their board had unequivocally stated cannabis use was of "no great threat" (Adams, 2016).

Regardless of the facts surrounding the benefits of cannabis, Anslinger pushed until the Marijuana Tax Law was enacted (Adams, 2016). The speculation that Mellon, Hearst and Dupont were involved in lobbying the federal government against cannabis because it threatened their empires in investments, paper and synthetic fibers interests has not been *thoroughly* substantiated [See Library of Congress for more details] (AP, 2015, Dunning, 2014 & The News Journal, 2015). But evidence is strong that between the timeframes of 1937 when the tax act was approved and 1942 when the federal government started a hard push for increased farming of hemp to replace foreign hemp supplies, that there was a concerted effort to put fear in the hearts of citizens regarding cannabis [4][5][6]. As to whether there would have been a net gain for the aforementioned individuals, the Mellon family did have pull within the Republican party (Wikipedia, 2018). But Andrew Mellon who served as US Secretary of Treasury had by 1932 left the position into private life, passing in 1937. Hearst was in his declining years by this point; in both popularity, wealth and health (Dunning, 2014 & Wikipedia, 2018). The DuPont family holdings might have had the most to gain, Rayon had already been in the marketplace for over a decade, and Nylon was patented by DuPont in 1937 (The News Journal, 2015 & Wikipedia, 2018). Several other discoveries from DuPont labs that had a profound effect on war cordage supplies for everything from blankets and parachute materials to jeep tires, and DuPont's added involvement in pharmaceuticals would see them as most able to gain (Dupont, 2014 & Wikipedia, 2018). The question remains was it for financial gain or the betterment of society? Further digging led me to an interesting viewpoint; associate professor at James Madison University Alan Levinovitz's studies regarding the relationship between religion and science (Brown, 2018). Levinovitz says there's a simple reason we look at sugar as evil: "throughout history, we've demonized the things we find hardest to resist (think of sexual pleasure in the Victorian times)" (Brown, 2018); the cannabis and sugar correlation is compelling.

- **When the Tide Turned**

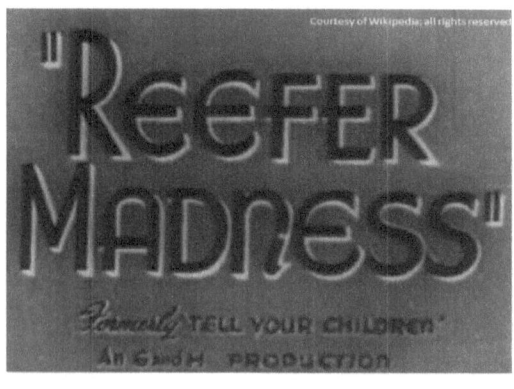

Tell Your Children (1936) the propaganda film that depicted cannabis as a tool to tear apart the very fabric of capitalism and democracy, was created by a church group in hopes of reinforcing stricter, more conservative moral codes. Since the repeal of the Volstead Act [Alcohol Prohibition] in 1933, it was the conservative opinion that our country's youth might fall to influences of drugs and alcohol that did not meet the moral majority's interests. The movie was branded and released across the country under multiple titles [6]. Some might say that ultimately, it was a successful attempt to keep America's power base firmly set (Adams, 2016), but it wasn't until 1969 that Anslinger's Marijuana Tax Act of 1937 was overturned; struck down as unconstitutional because having to purchase stamps to trade in cannabis, was finally recognized as self-incrimination (Anslinger, 1835-1975). The damage to the American consciousness was done however, and cannabis had become a noxious weed rather than being remembered as the healing plant it had been for centuries before around the globe. It was that same year [1969] President Richard Nixon placed the final coffin nail in cannabis by making sure that it was listed as a Schedule I drug, or being 'a narcotic having no medicinal

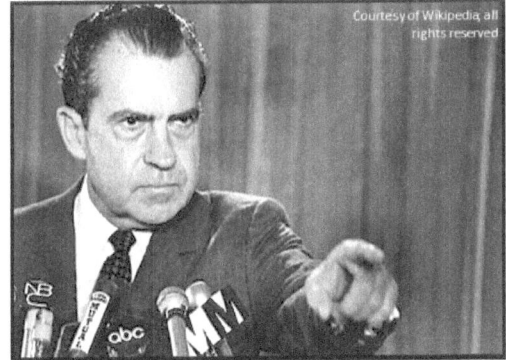

value'[6]. Four years later in 1973, Nixon established the Drug Enforcement Agency (DEA), and since then, the war on drugs has been a fixture in our culture and classrooms. More than a trillion dollars of taxpayer funds have been spent on the 'War on Drugs' over the last forty years. And while the question of cocaine, heroin and other narcotics and their management in society is beyond the scope of this book, demonizing and fighting a plant that throughout history in multiple industries and cultures has been successfully used to benefit mankind requires a long hard and objective look for other reasons (AP, 2015 & Brown, 2018). Are we truly better off having purposefully excluded this plant from medicine in our western methodologies? What could we have accomplished with even a portion of the trillion plus dollars that have been spent fighting cannabis; had we instead spent them on research and development. We can't fix the past, but it is time to find the true power of cannabis.

B: BRIEF CLARIFICATION; MARIJUANA OR HEMP?

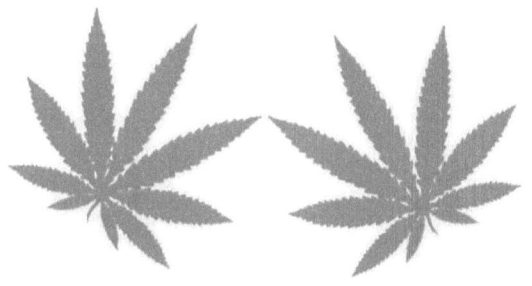

Marijuana and Hemp are more legal descriptions of cannabis than plant subspecies. Although C. Sativa and C. Indica, typically have slightly different leaf structures, and classically sativas are considered hemp plants, both C. Indica [Marijuana] and C. Sativa [Hemp] have been so hybridized over history as to create low and high THC plants in both categories (Wilder, 2016). No longer does a narrow leaf mean the plant is hemp and broad leaf mean the plant is full of psychoactive properties (Wilder, 2016). Less like the differences between Cavandish and Plantain bananas; the first eaten raw, while the latter is best cooked, and more the difference of male and female counterparts. Both have been used interchangeably for personal consumption and product manufacturing (Singh, 2017). C. Ruderalis, a possible third variety, is currently the Pluto of the cannabis world; it might be a third subspecies or might just be a type of C. Sativa; as of the writing of this book, the jury's still out [1]. What truly separates marijuana from hemp is only the percentage of the psychoactive *cannabinoid* THC found in the plant (Sawler et al, 2015). Both hemp and marijuana have THC as well as a host of other cannabinoid compounds; more than one hundred different molecules at last count, that make up the cannabinoid family. Only the notable psychoactive THC molecule or a derivative of THC is considered illegal by the Controlled Substances Act (Mead, 2016). Anything currently over .3% THC, and the plant is illegal by UN Narcotics Convention, and thus considered marijuana.

Fact: Hemp farmers have routinely over recent history had to destroy whole crops because THC levels tested above the .3% marker (NCSL, 2018).

Another interesting fact as we transition deeper into what cannabis does to us, the differences between activated and non-activated cannabis. THC and CBD, for instance, must be changed through heat or chemical process from their parent molecules; THCA and CBDA respectively. Tetrahydrocannabinolic Acid (THCA) and Cannabidiolic Acid (CBDA) naturally occur in cannabis but are not themselves psychoactive compounds [meaning they won't make you high] (DeVito & Staff, 2017). Their purpose, as we will read later, is to work specifically on pain and inflammation; just what you're looking for when it comes to topicals.

- **What are cannabinoids?**

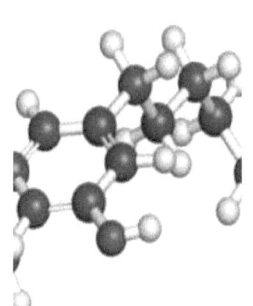

Cannabinoids are one of many of the compounds that exist within cannabis [and animals!]; molecules that act on a series of switches in our bodies known as neuro receptors. These switches are part of how our bodies interact with the world around us. All over our bodies, these neuro receptors react to chemicals, sending signals through a network that makes up the Endo Cannabinoid System (ECS) (DeVito, 2014, Janero & Makiyannis, 2014, Jacobs, 2017, Turcote et al, 2016, & Zou & Kumar, 2018). This complex system of chemical receptors found in *all* vertebrates assists in regulating the body's chemical and physical balance or *homeostasis* (DeVito,2017); from regulating appetite to fertility, cell lifespan and memory, and yes, even pain recognition and inflammation response (DeVito, 2017, Jacobs 2017, Janero & Makiyannis, 2014, National Academy of Sciences, 2017). Cannabinoids, like many other chemicals, have an impact on how our bodies perceive, function and interact with the world around us (Cascio et al, 2010). When molecules like THC meet the right receptors in our bodies, they effectively create the sensations we know as euphoria (Zou & Kumar, 2018). There are over 60 known cannabinoid types in any single cannabis plant (Brenneisen, 2007). But how did we get acquainted with cannabis? Normally, as with any other plant when foraging for food, there must be an attraction to it; whether because it smells good or interesting, or because through seeing someone or something else acting in a particular way [rabbits love to munch on cannabis], we decided to try and then realized a benefit. Or, we could speculate that it may have been something as simple as our early ancestors were trying to find a food to eat, or more likely, start a fire with some weeds near their camp [Let's be honest, would you want to eat anything that smelled like the southbound end of a northbound skunk without knowing what it does?]. Fire or food first, we will never know, but in either case, it would have been our sense of smell that helped bring cannabis into our lives (Paddock, 2018). By and of themselves, individual cannabinoids don't provide the total plant to mammal benefit that the cannabis plant has to offer, they would have been masked by odors (Russo, 2011); this is where *Terpenes* come in.

- Terpenes; How We Meet and Greet Our World

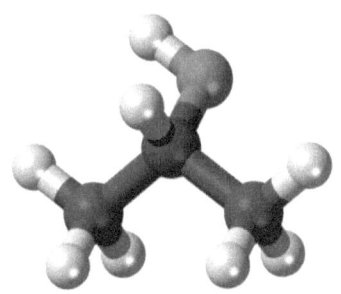

Our sense of smell and taste have guided our survival since our earliest days; enter Terpenes. Terpenes or Terpenoids are aromatic compounds found in *all* plant and animal life; designed to defend against predators or pathogens, while also attracting mates by conveying chemical messages; terpenes are a language all their own (Gershenzon & Dudareva, 2007). They are, in more general terms, the scents of life. Ever wonder why you feel a sense of calm when walking through a pine forest? You smell the Alpha and Beta Pinene all around you, which coincidentally are also found in parsley, dill, basil, rosemary, and yes, cannabis. What most people don't know is that beta-pinene is commonly used as an anti-depressant (Gershenzon & Dudareva, 2007). When we combine cannabinoids and terpenes from *any* source, a synergy or "Entourage Effect" occurs (Mechoulam, 1986); meaning the sum of the parts has a greater effect than any one component by itself. Myrcene, one of over 200 terpenes, and typically the most prevalent in cannabis, has a sedative effect that helps to amplify the effects of THC (Russo, 2011 & Mechoulam, 1986). But Myrcene is also found in oranges, hops, mangos, and lemongrass; just to name a few plants (Singh & Sharma, 2015). While terpenes are important in the chemistry of cannabis, they, like THC and CBD, are not the end all. Think of peanut butter and jelly sandwiches; each piece in the puzzle makes the whole better than the sum of its parts (Singh & Sharma, 2015).

- ECS: Enter CB1 & CB2 Receptors

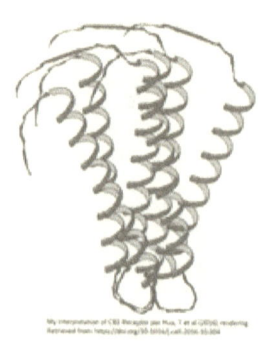

Artist's Rendering of CB1 Receptor (Hua et al, 2016)

We have three points of entry into our bodies; Inhalation [Lungs; via nose and mouth], Ingestion [Stomach/Intestines; via nose, mouth and other orifices], and Topical [Skin]. Of the three, topical is the most vulnerable, as it is our largest organ and most exposed to outside elements; which is why it is also the most protected. Without going into the specific details of how and why cannabis works, topically or otherwise, just know our bodies are reasonably good at gatekeeping; not allowing most foreign products entry into our bodies. A barrier created by specialized cells surrounding our smallest blood vessels (capillaries) acts as a filter, which is known as the blood/brain barrier (Chudler, 2017). Once cannabinoids get past these barriers and encounter two specific neuro receptors [that we're concerned with]; the receptors are triggered, and we feel the effects; These are known simply as CB1 and CB2 receptors.

Our endo cannabinoid system is made up of a variety of neuro receptors, which turn chemicals they meet into signals our bodies process to perform a variety of tasks. CB1 and CB2 receptors each accept and interact in specific ways with cannabinoids (Janero & Makiyannis, 2014). Although both receptor types are found throughout our bodies, CB1 receptors are found in larger concentrations in the brain and liver, while CB2 receptors are most frequently found in our gastrointestinal, skin, and immune systems (Janero & Makiyannis, 2014). Only CB1 receptors seem affected by THC, which is why we feel euphoria or anxiety in the brain when smoking or eating cannabis (Paddock, 2018). CB2 receptors have been found to regulate immune tissues, which affect inflammation and pain (Turcotte, C et al, 2016). Additional research has shown however that to get the best

overall effect for pain relief, THCA and CBDA (parent molecules) are required. They don't have to necessarily be a one to one ratio to work, because everyone's count of CB1 and CB2 receptors are different; just like a fingerprint.

Specifically, both compounds should be present to balance out each other's effects, in the same way as you might use one drug to combat pain, while another reduces inflammation (Baron et al, 2018, DeVito, 2014, Zou & Kumar, 2018). Terpenes work in concert with cannabinoids to enhance, or balance out the other's effects (Angus, 2017).

- It's Alphabet Soup...

THCA, THC, THCV, CBDA, CBD, CBN, CBG, CBV... The goal here isn't to prepare you for a degree in organic chemistry, but it is helpful to have a basic understanding and some facts surrounding how each of these affects you, so that you can make solid choices; *that will take some personal discovery, based on your willingness to try different products.* THC demonstrates analgesic, anti-emetic, and anti-inflammatory properties. CBD showed similar actions, plus anti-psychotic, anti-seizure, and anti-anxiety properties.

As previously stated, ratio requirements and effects differ for each person due to their CB receptor fingerprint; the number of both types of cannabinoid receptors in your body is what determines your personal limits. But we can offer typical ratio results for activated THC and CBD:

Table 1: Typical Responses to THC:CBD Ratios (Staff, 2017)	
THC: CBD Ratios	A: Typical Results B: Adverse Effects
1:0	A: High psychoactive effects; euphoria/mood change, & dizziness B: Tachycardia (racing heart), anxiety and paranoia
1:1	A: Psychoactive effect (lesser extent), CBD helps reduce risks. B: Increased CBD levels counteract THC; wakes you up more.
0:1	A: No mind-altering effects, inflammation decreases due to CBD B: Limited analgesic (pain killing) effect; CBD promotes wakefulness

The following list is a quick sample of some of the better-known cannabinoids; which I have dutifully named 'The Fab Seven'.

Table 2: The 'Fab 7' - Basic Cannabinoid Chart (Staff, 2017 & Tucker & Wikipedia, 2018)	
Molecule	*Name and specifics regarding effect, CB molecule, and receptor.*

CBG	**Cannabigerol** (non-psychoactive): The parent cannabinoid for all cannabinoids (THC, CBD, etc). Does influence serotonin receptors.
THCA	**Tetrahydrocannabonolic Acid** (Non-activated/Non-psychoactive): Parent molecule to THC that resides in cannabis' raw form. Relieves inflammation and pain; immune system regulator (CB1 receptors).
THC	**Tetrahydrocannabinol** (Psychoactive): Creates sense of euphoria, or anxiety in some users when inhaled or ingested; effect on serotonin; a neuro transmitter; [made by heating/aging THCA] (CB1 receptors).
CBDA	**Cannabidolic Acid** (Non-activated/non-psychoactive): Parent Molecule to CBD, also found in natural form. Inhibits cancer cell growth; Anti-inflammatory, anti-oxidant; similar to Omega-6 fatty acids (CB2 receptors).
CBD	**Cannabidiol** (non-psychoactive): Anti-Inflammatory, Anti-epileptic, anti-pain effects have been noted via ongoing research (CB2 Receptors).
CBN	**Cannabinol** (non-psychoactive): found in trace amounts in cannabis, mostly in degraded or aged cannabis. (CB1 and CB2 receptors).
CBV	**Cannabivarin** (non-psychoactive) Similar to CBN, it is an oxidized version of THCV

These are the primary cannabinoids you will be most likely to see when looking through products at your local dispensary. Where the previous chart referring to activated THC and CBD compounds are what is typically found in isolates, and vape pens, THCA, CBDA are the molecules most commonly associated with whole plant infused oils, topical solutions and flower that has not yet been heated, or *decarboxylized [decarbed]*.

FACT: Scientific findings corroborate that terpenes have a positive effect on Alzheimer's disease…the findings were published back in 1997 (Russo, 2011).

Table 3: Common Terpenes (Gershenzon & Dudareva, 2007 & Russo, 2011)	
This list is only a sample of the vast list of terpenoids in the plant and animal family; and just a few from the cannabis plant. There are other terpenoids outside of the cannabis species that can and do add a synergistic effect to its beneficial abilities.	
Terpene	**Effect**
Cannabis-related	
Myrcene	Sedative; amplifies effect of THC (Musty et al, 1976)
Linalool	Anti-convulsant (Hill et al, 2010), helps with burns (Qin et al, 2008), muscle relaxant (Kavia et al, 2010), Anti-anxiety (Russo et al, 2005), Alzheimer's disease (Volicer et al, 1997; Eubanks et al, 2006)
Pinene	Effective against MRSA (Appendino et al, 200*), Bronchodilator (Williams et al, 1976), Muscle relaxant (Kavia et al, 2010), Alzheimer's disease inhibitor (Volicer et al, 1997; Eubanks et al, 2006)
β-caryophyllene	Anti-hyperalgesic (Bolognini et al, 2010)
Limonene	Breast cancer resistance protein (Holland et al, 2008), Anti-depressant (Musty & Deyo, 2006), Antioxidant (Hampson et al, 1998), Alzheimer's disease (Volicer et al, 1997; Eubanks et al, 2006), and muscle relaxant (Kavia et al, 2010)
Caryophyllene Oxide	Anti-fungal (ElSohly et al, 1982), TRPM8 antagonist; helps with prostate cancer (De Petrocellis et al, 2011)
Nerolidol	Similar to Myrcene, Sedative (Musty et al, 1976)
Phytol	GABA uptake inhibitor; anti-convulsant (Banerjee et al, 1975)
Other non-cannabis plant related examples of terpenes	
Mentha Piperita (Peppermint)	Liver & Kidney benefits, reduces inflammation (Bellasoued et al, 2018 & Staff, WebMD, 2018)

Eucalyptol (Eucalyptus)	Enhances memory/mood, anti-inflammatory, anticancer, promotes normal cell function (Khan et al, 2014)
Carvacrol (Oregano)	Antibacterial, antiviral, antifungal properties (Rowles, 2017)
Vanillin (*Not Synthetic*)	Antioxidant, antibacterial (Group, 2014) *Ethyl vanillin;* use caution; can irritate lungs/gut [see reference] (Sky, 2017).

The nice thing about terpenes, is that since they are found in all plants and animals in nature; oils can be *carefully* chosen and added to cannabis products to improve a product's overall performance; where an individual cannabis strain might be lacking, or just need an extra boost to create a discrete aroma change.

FACT: terpenes are small enough on their own to break through the blood brain barrier; which is why smells and taste responses are so immediate.

Here are some examples of additional essential oils that are currently used in the industry to supplement cannabis products; with a word of caution on each...

Table 4: Typical Essential Oils Used in Topicals	
Oil	Use & Effects
Lemongrass	Is antibacterial, stress, anxiety, depression reliever; also thought to relieve pain and swelling, reduce fever. *Not recommended to be taken by mouth; undiluted oil taken internally may be fatal.*
Camphor	*; undiluted oil taken internally may be fatal.*
Peppermint	Used for common cold, cough, inflammation, heartburn,

	nausea, IBS, helps with kidney and liver issues (Bellassoued et al & Staff, WebMD, 2018)
Lavender	Helps with anxiety used topically or in aromatherapy. Known to cause breast development in children near puberty. Do not take by mouth (Roach, 2017). Similar results seen in tea tree and soy, as these are all sources of phytoestrogens (WebMD, 2018).
Eucalyptus	Natural antiseptic, anti-inflammatory, and antibacterial; highly effective in treating wounds, bug bites, minor cuts, acne. Research showing benefits in Alzheimer's & cancer treatment in small doses; *caution undiluted oil can be fatal, don't take internally*. Enhances memory and normal cell function (apoptosis) (Khan et al, 2014).
Citrus	Antioxidant, antibacterial, immune system support. May cause skin sensitivity in sunlight if applied topically.
Cumin	Helps with allergies, asthma, diabetes, boost immune system, and more. Safe to eat but can cause blisters applied topically.
Capsaicin	Is shown to help relieve pain; by blocking pain messages to your nerves. It can help with joint conditions, Fibromyalgia, muscle sprains, migraines, neuropathy; use in diluted form. Undiluted, capsaicin is also used by law enforcement as a formidable deterrent.

Typically, the following essential oils are added in small amounts to topicals, to improve the entourage effect (Staff, 2017). Considered as safe to use, most should only be added in small amounts to keep from causing harm either due to concentration levels, or simply due to possible toxic reaction. The following list is by no means complete, but it does show an example of how these terpenes can increase the benefits of cannabis use…or make them worse if not done properly. [See 'final notes' for further information].

C: CONSUMPTION
CHOICES & DECISIONS

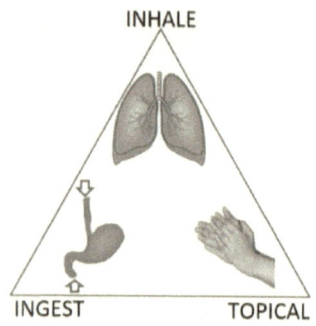

Research is constantly ongoing, but what has been shown already is scientifically ground-breaking. Our bodies receptors use our sense of smell and taste to help effect whole body change and balance (Baron et al, 2018 & Booth et al, 2017). Since there are so many combinations of cannabinoids and terpenes available from a variety of plant and those that can be added to improve synergy, it means our bodies have multiple ways of using cannabis and other plants. With CB1 and CB2 receptors all over our bodies, the question remains, *what is our goal with cannabis use, and what is the most efficient method, based on the need?* We have already covered the three ways in which cannabinoids and terpenes can be used; through inhaling, ingestion or topical application (See Cannabis Use Chart). What we haven't covered is the product types, or the immediacy of effect and response. Some people prefer smoking or vaping, others choose edibles, suppositories, or other bodily insertables; still more prefer topicals, or a mix.

- **Inhaling Cannabis**

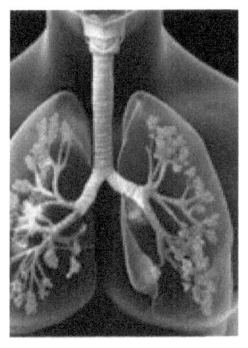

From an objective standpoint, burning of any product and inhaling it, no matter how good you are told it is for you, is going to leave micro particulates in your lungs; oil or flower [smoke; even through a bong, just has tinier particles debris] (Staff, 2014). It will over time, cause lung scaring just like any other inhaled pollutant; bong or no (Staff, 2014). But ultimately knowing that is a distinct possibility allows you to make an informed choice as an adult. Smoking or vaping, which burns oil and allows inhalation, is a quick and simple way to reach the desired effect to the head and body, but usually doesn't last as long as ingesting (See Generic Use Chart).

- Ingesting Cannabis,

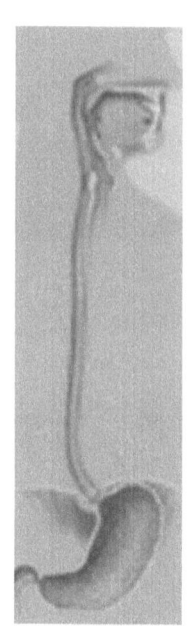

Whether consuming or using insertables, ingesting is another means of using cannabis. Edibles can come in the form of dressings, cooking oils, candies, or tinctures to name a few. Insertables also come in different forms; suppositories, tampons and even sex toys, designed to deliver a full dosage of activated and non-activated cannabinoids; whether for pain relief or pleasure, this method takes longer to affect the body, because the cannabinoids must first be absorbed and processed through internal organs; intestines, and liver, rather than going right into the bloodstream and straight to the brain. The lungs deliver in mere seconds, but the results of edibles last longer. Typically, edibles are where micro-dosing really comes into play. But If too much is consumed at once in either method and you are not prepared, the resulting effect may leave you stuck in a chair waiting for the effects to wear off; known as couchlock (Renee, 2005).

The common recommendation is to start with small amounts, allowing time to feel the full impact before increasing dosage.

- **Topical Application**

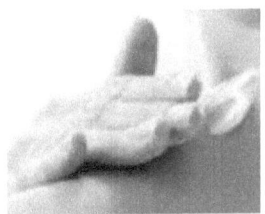

Topicals; lotions, slaves, transdermal patches, soaking salts, anything applied to the skin, is usually designed for specific area relief; whereas the previous two methods are designed for a whole-body experience (Reiman, 2014). Topicals typically should use non-activated cannabinoids and terpene combinations infused into carrier oils or other solutions to treat pain in specific areas of the body [Unless using transdermal patches] (Reiman, 2014). Topicals are perfect for the individual that wants to just take care of pain and stay alert, without the interest of getting high.

Per Reiman, transdermal patches may cause positive urinalysis tests, whereas other topicals normally will not; unless applied over broken skin where the solution may enter the bloodstream (2014).

Smoking/vaping results usually wear off approximately 20 minutes after usage stops; depending on strain strength. Edibles start and end slower, where topical effects can and often do last all day. Regardless of your method of choice, if you are still not sure, review the above chart, then ask your local budtender.

Cannabis Product Generic Use Chart							
		Psychoactive		Want more detailed information? Ask your budtender for a copy of 'The ABC's of THCBD' or visit skunksbutt.com			
Use	Type	CBD only	THC/CBD	Initial Effect	High	Lasts	Used for	Test Positive?
Inhale	Smoke	No	Yes	Immediate	Head/Body	1/2 - 2 hours, depending on amount/strength	Head/Whole body experience using joints, bongs, or vape pens	Yes*
	Vape		Yes					
Ingest	Edible	No	Yes	<30 min.	Head/Body	Several Hours	Whole body experience: Cooking oils, Salad dressings, Candies/Cookies, Suppositories, Other insertables, etc.	Yes*
	Insert		Yes					
Topical	Apply	No	No	1 - 5 min.	Body	Varies; 2 - 12 hours	Blocks specific area pain. Roll-ons, salves, creams, bath salts; good for joints & muscles; back, hip, knees, feet & hands	No**

* Unless CBD only. Must have less than .3% THC to be considered hemp, and thus not register on urinalysis. Results vary person to person
** Transdermal patches have been shown to cause positive test results, otherwise topicals typically are safe. Results vary person to person

All three types of *cannabis use* have been shown helpful for Migraines, Tremors, Epilepsy, Fibromyalgia, Cerebral Palsy, Cancer cell inhibition. Over 20,000 medical & scientific studies have been performed to date proving benefits.

FINAL NOTE
THE ADDITIVE BENEFITS F ESSENTIAL OILS

Remember our earlier discussion regarding the synergies of cannabis and terpenes, and how terpenes are found in every plant? Let's go back to the example of the peanut butter and jelly sandwich. PBnJ sandwiches are good (provided of course you don't have a peanut allergy; if so, then stick to almonds…peanuts are not a nut, but a legume; so they are not the same), but do they taste the same on white bread as on cracked wheat; or rye? How about the difference between grape and blackberry jelly? Every time you add or remove an ingredient, it has an effect of changing the texture, flavors, and ultimately the experience, thus product effectiveness. When dealing with terpenes in topicals, edibles, oils or flower, they play an integral role in how well the product works (Paddock, 2018). Ever use Vicks Vapo-rub on your chest when you had a stuffy head? The terpenes associated with

Eucalyptus, Camphor, Menthol and a host of other ingredients are what helped to make you feel better. A word of caution should you decide to make your own compounds. ***Study your essential oils***; their benefits and side effects before mixing up a batch. There is a saying for mushroom collectors that bears learning:

'Essential' Words of Wisdom

There are old mushroom pickers,
There are bold mushroom pickers;
But very few old, bold, mushroom pickers.
- Old Picker [Anon]

1. How much synergy is too much?
2. What if I'm allergic to an ingredient, and it's not listed?

- Terpenes (& Essential Oils); natures response to fight or flight

Essential Oils should be handled with care, especially in their concentrated form. Many are toxic, even fatal unless properly diluted in a carrier oil (coconut, almond, grapeseed or other). It takes time and practice to get combinations and dosages just right when mixing topicals; a great deal of study and practice to know what mixes well, what doesn't, and what should be totally avoided. Understand that when you purchase *any* topicals, cannabis or otherwise, it is important to read the ingredients list to verify whether you may have medical concerns. Any product that doesn't give you full disclosure of ingredients might be one to give a second thought about before using. Why? *What if you have allergies and can't tell what's in the product?* 'Proprietary blends' or a product that masks its ingredients might be one to shy away from unless you can get full disclosure from the manufacturer; even if they mention "products are GRAS rated" (GRAS stands for Generally Recognized As Safe), there are still ingredients generally listed as safe for consumption that can cause harm (Dolan et al, 2010). Sage oil is a great example. Many people really enjoy having sausage in the morning, but sage essential oil is not recommended as an additive to massage oils; it contains a terpene called Beta Thujone which can cause central nervous system damage and kidney failure (Dolan et al, 2010). Beta Thujone was a main reason Absinthe was made illegal in the U.S. back in the early 1900's (Dolan et al, 2010). It has high levels of Beta-Thujone that comes from wormwood; used to cure or flavor the drink. Lavender and soy are another example of possible problem oils that are used extensively; the phytoestrogen or plant estrogen compounds have been found to change breast size in males as well as females (Pathak, 2017). So, does this mean you'll drop dead from eating sausage, or using a topical with sage oil in it? The cholesterol and salt in the sausage are more likely to do damage, unless allergic, than the sage oil in your product; like everything else, it's always about concentration in the product, or how much and how highly concentrated the essential oils are in the carrier product it is mixed in that determines possible damage; it comes down to trust. Ultimately, it is always in the manufacturer's best interest to carefully blend their products to keep their customers safe. That being said, I prefer *knowing and researching* what is in my products. Companies that wish to keep their ingredients secret can still list all items while keeping their processing methods and/or percentages private; that way their customers can feel secure because they are informed, and companies are looking out for everyone's welfare; both sides win.

- **Summary of ABC's**

We covered a lot of information in this book. Your takeaway should be as follows:

1. Cannabis has been used and recommended by the medical community for longer than any of our current forms of government have been around to stigmatize

them. Cannabis is a respectable medicine with true benefit that is finally coming back into its own.

2. We all learn by two methods; studying (or modeling) and doing. Hopefully this book will get you interested in reading more about the benefits of cannabis and its history. Then, if interested and you are a *consenting* adult, trying some products (in small doses first); remembering what your goal is:

   a. **For a head/body high**, micro-dose *activated* THC/CBD products; inhalable or ingestible

   b. **To get a whole-body experience**, use combined *non-activated* THCA and CBDA products

   c. **To relieve local/specific pain**, use THCA/CBDA topicals

3. Cannabinoids and terpenes work best in conjunction. Yes, you can still get high from THC isolates, and can get some pain relief from CBD-only oils, but if you are looking for the full beneficial effects of cannabis, stick with crafted whole-plant products; otherwise, you're just blowing smoke.

REFERENCES
AND ADDITIONAL READING SUGGESTIONS

AACM. (2018). Suggested Resource Links. American Academy of Cannabinoid Medicine. Retrieved from: http://aacmsite.org/suggested-resource-links/

Abel, E. (1980). Marijuana - The First Twelve Thousand Years. Schaffer Library of Drug Policy. Retrieved from: http://www.druglibrary.org/schaffer/hemp/history/first12000/abel.htm#intro

Adams, C. (2016). [Harry Anslinger] The man behind the marijuana ban for all
the wrong reasons. CBS News. Retrieved from: https://www.cbsnews.com/news/harry-anslinger-the-man-behind-the-marijuana-ban/

Angus, C, (2017). Some of the Parts: Is Marijuana's "Entourage Effect" Scientifically Valid? Scientific American. Retrieved from: https://www.scientificamerican.com/article/some-of-the-parts-is-marijuana-rsquo-s-ldquo-entourage-effect-rdquo-scientifically-valid/

Anslinger, H. (1835-1975). H.J. Anslinger papers, 1835-1975. Penn State University Libraries. Retrieved from: https://www.libraries.psu.edu/findingaids/1875.htm

AP. (2015). War on Drugs. Associated Press. Retrieved from: https://www.foxnews.com/world/ap-impact-after-40-years-1-trillion-us-war-on-drugs-has-failed-to-meet-any-of-its-goals

Baron, E., Lucas P., Eades, J., Hogue, O. (2018). Patterns of medicinal cannabis use, strain analysis, and substitution effect among patients with migraine, headache, arthritis, and chronic pain in a medicinal cannabis cohort. US National Library of Medicine National Institutes of Health. Retrieved from: https://www.ncbi.nlm.nih.gov/pmc/articles/PMC5968020/

Bellassoued, K., Hsouna, A. Athmouni, K.,Pelt, J.,Ayadi, F., Rebai, T., Elfeki, A. (2018). Protective effects of Mentha piperita L. leaf essential oil…US National Library of Medicine. Retrieved from: https://www.ncbi.nlm.nih.gov/pmc/articles/PMC5761127/

Booth, J., Page, J., Bohlmann, J. (2017). Terpene Synthases from Cannabis sativa. US National Library of Medicine National Institutes of Health. Retrieved from: https://www.ncbi.nlm.nih.gov/pmc/articles/PMC5371325/

Brenneisen, R. (2007). Chemistry and Analysis of Phytocannabinoids and Other Cannabis Constituents. Medicinal Genomics. Retrieved from: https://www.medicinalgenomics.com/wp-content/uploads/2011/12/Chemical-constituents-of-cannabis.pdf

Brown, J. (2018). Is sugar really bad for you? BBC. Retrieved from: http://www.bbc.com/future/story/20180918-is-sugar-really-bad-for-you

Burke, A. (2016). How Long Do Dogs Live? American Kennel Club. Retrieved from: https://www.akc.org/expert-advice/health/how-long-do-dogs-live/

CABI. (2017). Invasive Species Compendium. CABI. Retrieved from: https://www.cabi.org/isc/datasheet/14497

Cascio, MG., Gauson, L., Stevenson, LA, Ross, RA., and Pertwee, RG. (2010). Evidence that the plant cannabinoid cannabigerol is a highly potent a2-adrenoceptor agonist and moderately potent 5HT1A receptor antagonist. US National Library of Medicine. National Institutes of Health. Retrieved from: https://www.ncbi.nlm.nih.gov/pmc/articles/PMC2823359/

Chudler, E. (2017). The Blood Brain Barrier. University of Washington. Retrieved from: https://faculty.washington.edu/chudler/bbb.html

Dept of Agriculture (Producer). (1942). Hemp for Victory [Movie]. Wikipedia. Video file: https://upload.wikimedia.org/wikipedia/commons/3/33/Hemp_for_Victory_1942.webm

DeVito, L. (2017). CB1 and CB2: Different Cannabinoid Receptors in the Brain. Labroots. Retrieved from: https://www.labroots.com/trending/health-and-medicine/7420/cb1-cb2-cannabinoid-receptors-brain

Dolan, L., Matulka, R., Burdock, G. (2010). Naturally Occurring Food Toxins. Retrieved from: https://www.ncbi.nlm.nih.gov/pmc/articles/PMC3153292/

Dunning, B. (2014). Hemp, Hearst, and Prohibition. Skeptoid. Retrieved from: https://skeptoid.com/episodes/4401

Dupont. (2014). Dupont Phoenix Heritage. DuPont. Retrieved from: http://www2.dupont.com/Phoenix_Heritage/en_US/1906_b_detail.html

Dvorak, J. (2018). The History of Hemp in America. CBDOiled. Retrieved from: http://www.hemphasis.net/History/harriedhemp.htm

Encyclopedia Britannica (2018). Du Pont Family. Encyclopedia Britannica. Retrieved from: https://www.britannica.com/topic/DuPont-Company

Gershenzon, J., Dudareva, N., (2007). The function of terpene natural products in the natural world. Nature Chemical Biology. Retrieved from: https://www.nature.com/articles/nchembio.2007.5

Grant, M. (2018). The trick to learning when to cut your losses. BBC.org. Retrieved from:

http://www.bbc.com/capital/story/20180914-the-trick-to-learning-when-to-cut-your-losses

Group, E. (2014). What is Vanillin? Global Healing Center. Retrieved from: https://www.globalhealingcenter.com/natural-health/vanillin/

Haze, N. (2018). How Long Does It Take to Grow Weed Indoors? Grow Weed Easy.com. Retrieved from: https://www.growweedeasy.com/how-long-does-it-take-to-grow-weed

Hirst, K. (2018). Plant Domestication. ThoughtCo. Retrieved from: https://www.thoughtco.com/plant-domestication-table-dates-places-170638

Jacobs, M. (2017). Cannabinoids and Terpenes; What is the Difference? Terpenes and Testing Magazine. Retrieved from: https://terpenesandtesting.com/cannabinoids-terpenes-difference/

Janero, D. Makiyannis, A. (2014). Terpenes and Lipids of the Endocannabinoid and Transient-Receptor-Potential-Channel Biosignaling Systems. US National Library of Medicine. Retrieved from: https://www.ncbi.nlm.nih.gov/pmc/articles/PMC4948289/

Khan, A., Vaibhav, K., Javed, H., Tabassum, R., Ahmed, M., Khan, M.M., Khan, M.B., Shrivastava, P., Islam, F., Siddiqui, M., Safhi, M., Islam, F., (2014). 1,8-Cineole (Eucalyptol) Mitigates Inflammation in Amyloid Beta Toxicated PC12 Cells…
Springer. Retrieved from: https://link.springer.com/article/10.1007/s11064-013-1231-9

Klabunde, R. (2013). Alpha-Adrenoceptor Agonists. Cardiovascular Pharmacology Concepts. Retrieved from: https://www.cvpharmacology.com/vasoconstrictor/alpha-agonist

Klein T.W., Newton C.A. (2007) Therapeutic Potential of Cannabinoid-Based Drugs. In: Shurin M.R., Smolkin Y.S.
(eds) Immune-Mediated Diseases. Advances in Experimental Medicine and Biology, vol 601. Springer, New York, NY. Retrieved from: https://link.springer.com/chapter/10.1007/978-0-387-72005-0_43

Lafrance, A. (2015). Was Marijuana Really Less Potent in the 1960's? The Atlantic. Retrieved from: https://www.theatlantic.com/technology/archive/2015/03/was-marijuana-really-less-potent-in-the-1960s/387010/

Laws. (2017). Understanding the 18th Amendment. Laws. Retrieved from: https://constitution.laws.com/american-history/constitution/constitutional-amendments/18th-amendment

McNearney, A. (2018). The Complicated History of Cannabis in the US. History. Retrieved from: https://www.history.com/news/marijuana-criminalization-reefer-madness-history-flashback

Mead, J. (2016). The legal status of cannabis (marijuana) and cannabidiol (CBD) under U.S. law. ScienceDirect. Retrieved from: https://www.sciencedirect.com/science/article/pii/S1525505016305856

Miller, S. (2017). IS Cannabis Really More Potent Today Than It Was 20 Years Ago? Origin Cannabis. Retrieved from: https://www.originscannabis.com/marijuana-potency/

National Academy of Sciences. (2017). The Health Effects of Cannabis and Cannabinoids: The Current State of Evidence and Recommendations
for Research. National Institutes of Health. Retrieved from: https://www.ncbi.nlm.nih.gov/books/NBK425762/

NCSL. (2018). National Conference of State Legislatures. Retrieved from: http://www.ncsl.org/research/agriculture-and-rural-development/state-industrial-hemp-statutes.aspx

Oberhaus, D. (2016). This is the First Atomic-Level Image of the Weed Receptors in your Brain. Motherboard.
Retrieved from: https://motherboard.vice.com/en_us/article/8q8k8z/atomic-level-image-of-the-weed-receptors

Paddock, C. (2018). Olfactory receptors 'do more than smell'. Medical News Today. Retrieved from: https://www.medicalnewstoday.com/articles/322507.php

Pathak, N (2017). What are Essential Oils? WebMD. Retrieved from: https://www.webmd.com/skin-problems-and-treatments/ss/slideshow-essential-oils

Reiman, A. PhD (2014). I Use Medical Marijuana in Topical Form… Drug Policy Alliance. Retrieved from: http://www.drugpolicy.org/blog/i-use-medical-marijuana-topical-form-pain-will-i-test-positive-drug-test

Renee, C. (2005). Couchlock [definition]. Urban Dictionary. Retrieved from: https://www.urbandictionary.com/define.php?term=couchlock

Reynolds, P. (2015). Medicinal Cannabis: The Evidence. BMJ. Retrieved from: https://www.bmj.com/sites/default/files/response_attachments/2015/03/Medicinal%20Cannabis%20The%20Evidence%20V1.pdf

Roach, K. (2017). Your Good Health: Lavender oil is still a drug, with side-effects. Times Colonist. Retrieved from: https://www.timescolonist.com/life/health/your-good-health-lavender-oil-is-still-a-drug-with-side-effects-1.21186237

Rowles, A. (2017). 9 Benefits and Uses of Oregano Oil. Healthline. Retrieved from: https://www.healthline.com/nutrition/9-oregano-oil-benefits-and-uses

Russo, E. (2011). Taming THC: potential cannabis synergy and phytocannabinoid-terpenoid entourage effects. British Journal of Pharmacology. Retrieved from: https://www.ncbi.nlm.nih.gov/pmc/articles/PMC3165946/

Saletan, W. (2005). FrankenFido Our Creepiest genetic invention; the dog. Human Nature. Retrieved from: http://www.slate.com/articles/health_and_science/human_nature/2005/12/frankenfido.html

Sandoiu, A (2018). Newly found organ may lead to 'dramatic advances'. Medical News Today. Retrieved from: https://www.medicalnewstoday.com/articles/321344.php?iacp

Schaffer Library (2006). Schaffer Library of Drug Policy. Drug Library. Retrieved from: http://www.druglibrary.net/toc.htm

Singh, B. & Sharma, R. (2015). Plant terpenes: defense responses, phylogenetic analysis, regulation and clinical applications. NCBI. Retrieved from: https://www.ncbi.nlm.nih.gov/pmc/articles/PMC4362742/

Singh, A. (2017). Can marijuana be made into cloth... Quora. Retrieved from: https://www.quora.com/Can-marijuana-be-made-into-cloth-rope-paper-etc-like-hemp-Can-you-get-high-by-smoking-hemp

Sky, Z. (2017). Ethyl vanillin – toxicity, side effects, diseases and environmental impacts. Chemical News. Retrieved from: http://chemicals.news/2017-12-05-ethyl-vanillin-toxicity-side-effects-diseases-and-environmental-impacts.html

Staff, Cannabis. (2014). Water pipes, 'bongs' and 'hookahs': What does the evidence say about harms? Cannabis Information & Support. Retrieved from: https://cannabissupport.com.au/workplace-and-clinical-resources/publications/bulletins/water-pipes-bongs-and-hookahs-what-does-the-evidence-say-about-harms/

Staff, CrescoLabs. (2018). What is THCA? CrescoLabs. Retrieved from: https://www.crescolabs.com/cannabinoids/thca/

Staff, Green Leaf. (2018). Cannabinoid Receptors 101: Why Do We Have Them? Green Leaf. Retrieved from: https://www.greenrelief.ca/blog/cannabinoid-receptors/
Staff. (2018). World War Two Timeline. History on the Net. Retrieved from: https://www.historyonthenet.com/world-war-2-timeline-2/

Staff, Leaf Science. (2017). Marijuana and the Entourage Effect. Leaf Science. Retrieved from: https://www.leafscience.com/2017/12/08/marijuana-entourage-effect/

Staff, MedicalJane. (2016). How many terpenes are in cannabis?

MedicalJane. Retrieved from: https://www.medicaljane.com/question/how-many-terpenes-are-in-weed/

Staff, UPG. (2017). THC-A and CBD-A: What are the Benefits? United Patients Group. Retrieved from: https://unitedpatientsgroup.com/blog/2017/01/19/thca-and-cbda-what-are-the-benefits/

Staff, WebMD. (2018). Peppermint. WebMD. Retrieved from: https://www.webmd.com/vitamins/ai/ingredientmono-705/peppermint

Staff, Zamnesia. (2017). The Benefits of Different CBD:THC Ratios. Zamnesia. Retrieved from: https://www.zamnesia.com/blog-the-benefits-of-different-cbd-thc-ratios-n1323

The News Journal. (2015). DuPont Timeline. Delaware Online. Retrieved from: https://www.delawareonline.com/story/news/2015/12/11/dupont-timeline/77156628/

Tucker, A. (2018). Why Pot makes you Paranoid – But Mellows Out Your Buddies. Men's Health. Retrieved from: https://www.menshealth.com/about/a19038260/why-pot-makes-you-paranoid-but-mellows-out-your-buddies/

Turcote et al, (2016). The CB2 receptor and its role as a regulator of inflammation. US National Library of Medicine. Retrieved from: https://www.ncbi.nlm.nih.gov/pmc/articles/PMC5075023/

[2] USDA (Producer). Evans, R. (Director). (1942). Hemp for Victory. Retrieved from: https://en.wikipedia.org/wiki/Hemp_for_Victory.

Voeks, R. (2014). Cannabis: Evolution and Ethnobotany. Taylor Francis. Retrieved from: https://www.tandfonline.com/doi/full/10.1080/2325548X.2014.901859?scroll=top&needAccess=true

WebMD. (2018). Lemongrass. WebMD. Retrieved from: https://www.webmd.com/vitamins/ai/ingredientmono-719/lemongrass

Wikipedia. (2018). Andrew Mellon. Wikipedia.
Retrieved from: https://en.wikipedia.org/wiki/Andrew_Mellon

Wikipedia. (2018). Bureau of Prohibition. Wikipedia.
Retrieved from: https://en.wikipedia.org/wiki/Bureau_of_Prohibition

[1] Wikipedia, (2018). Cannabis. Wikipedia.
Retrieved from: https://en.wikipedia.org/wiki/Cannabis

[3] Wikipedia, (2018). Cannabidiol. Wikipedia.
Retrieved from: https://en.wikipedia.org/wiki/Cannabidiol

[7] Wikipedia. (2018). DuPont. Wikipedia. Retrieved from: https://en.wikipedia.org/wiki/DuPont

[4] Wikipedia, (2018). Legal history of cannabis in the United States. Retrieved from: https://en.wikipedia.org/wiki/Legal_history_of_cannabis_in_the_United_States

[5] Wikipedia (2018). Temperance Movement. Wikipedia. Retrieved from: https://en.wikipedia.org/wiki/Temperance_movement

[6] Wikipedia. (2018). War on Drugs. Wikipedia.
Retrieved from: https://en.wikipedia.org/wiki/War_on_drugs
[8] Wikipedia. (2018). List of Wars 1900-1944. Wikipedia. Retrieved from: https://en.wikipedia.org/wiki/List_of_wars_1900%E2%80%931944

Wilcox, B. (2018). The Effects of THCA and CBDA on The Human Endocannabinoid System. CAT Scientific. Retrieved from: https://www.catscientific.com/effects-thca-cbda-human-endocannabinoid-system/

ABOUT THE AUTHOR

Douglas is a polymath; has enjoyed working in multiple careers throughout his life to include the U.S. military, 9-1-1 (Network & computer systems), consulting in web applications & computer services, and the cannabis industry (once legalized in Oregon). His degrees include an AAS in Airframe Metals Technology, a Bachelor's of Science in Human Resources Management and his Master's degree in Business Administration. He lives with his wife, children and grandchildren in Willamette Valley Oregon

www.ingramcontent.com/pod-product-compliance
Lightning Source LLC
Chambersburg PA
CBHW030514220526
45464CB00006B/2785